the first year of
the rest of your
life

the first year of
the rest of your
life

reflections for survivors of breast cancer

charla hudson honea, editor

The Pilgrim Press
Cleveland, Ohio

The Pilgrim Press, Cleveland, Ohio 44115

© 1997 by The Pilgrim Press

Printed in the United States of America on acid-free paper

02 01 00 99 98 97   5 4 3 2 1

Library of Congress Cataloging-in-Publication Data
    The first year of the rest of your life : reflections for survivors of breast cancer / edited by Charla Hudson Honea.
        p.   cm.
    ISBN 0-8298-1209-1 (pbk. : alk. paper)
    1. Breast—Cancer—Patients—Biography.   I. Honea, Charla.
RC280.B8F56   1997
362.1'9699449—dc21
[B]   97-25949
                                                          CIP

For all women whose lives are touched by breast cancer.

The distinguished poet Maya Angelou once wrote that "being a woman is hard work....The woman who survives intact and happy must be at once tender and tough." I could not agree with her more. Being a woman with responsibilities, goals, and dreams is hard work. It is with hope and humor—the things for which we lean on each other—that we fortify ourselves.

I first learned this lesson through the experience of my sister, Susan G. Komen. Suzy was diagnosed with breast cancer at the tender age of thirty-three. It was 1975 and treatment options were a great deal more limited than they are today. Suzy sought treatment first from her local physician and ultimately from a team at M.D. Anderson in Houston, Texas. During her battle, she endured chemotherapy, radiation, and numerous operations. She saw her body change and grow weak. I watched her go through it all. When the load became almost too heavy to carry, Suzy was the one to lift me and my family with her grace and humor. At every turn, she found something to smile about. She was constantly filled with hope for the future. Her spirit never sagged. I admired her for the abundance of life she carried within her. Even as we sat in the waiting rooms of hospitals, Suzy thought of others. She said to me, "As soon as I get better, let's do something about this. You can do something to speed up the research. I know you can. And I want to fix up this waiting room and make it pretty for the women who have to be here. This isn't right."

After three years of fierce determination, Suzy lost her battle with cancer. But before she died, she asked me to carry out her wish to help other women confronted with the disease.

At first I lay awake at night wondering how I could help other women. How could I make a difference? How could one voice be heard?

I wanted to do something to keep my sister's memory alive. So in 1982 I formed the Susan G. Komen Breast Cancer Foundation. Then in 1984 I found a lump in my own breast. I had not imagined what it would be like to hear those words "It's cancer" referring to my own body. But that is what happened.

Fortunately, I had more information and options than Suzy. And my experience strengthened my passion and commitment to the organization. Today Suzy's foundation is a leader in the field of breast cancer research funding, education, and legislative advocacy. I have learned—from my sister and from the many women I meet in my work—that hope is the key. I have seen women in their most despondent moments receive hope by watching other women who have survived. I have seen women who once feared loss of their femininity gain confidence by sharing their experience with another.

From each of these encounters, I have witnessed the best and the worst of coping with cancer. My life is richer and fuller now and I appreciate the value of good health as never before. I'm not the first woman to have dealt with breast cancer. But I know that when a woman is first diagnosed and is facing treatment, she often feels as if no one understands. *The First Day of the Rest of Your Life* can be a wonderful antidote to this feeling. I am touched by the courage and hope contained in each of the stories in this fine book. These stories remind us that shared feelings— from sorrow to triumph—can reach out and teach those who may be at the start of our already traveled path. I am reminded of how I felt before I formed Suzy's foundation, even before I conceived of it. I wondered about the impact of one person, one voice. The women in this book, more than seventy-five individual voices, most likely felt the same way. However, their contribution to *The First Day of the Rest of Your Life* illustrates how one voice attracts another to the hope. I think anyone who reads these remembrances will be enriched and inspired. You will meet Kim who states that "cancer does make it even more important to be your own self." And you will read that Lee says, "There are a lot of things I wish I had done in the past. Well, I've been given a second chance and I'm going to use it!"

I am deeply touched by how these wonderful women, facing this difficult disease, are "at once tender and tough." It is within their spirit and courage that real hope may be found.

Nancy Brinker

When I was in college in the sixties, the word "trip" was used quite a bit. It usually referred to an experience of some kind, often fun or exciting. It could also mean an experience that was complicated or amazing or difficult to explain. Whether the experience was negative or positive, you might hear someone exclaim, "What a trip!" As I sat down to write this introduction, I recalled that phrase somewhat wistfully—a strong reminder of a relatively innocent and more carefree time. Then I realized how appropriate that phrase is for me when I consider my own experience with breast cancer. In that process I have experienced all the varied interpretations of the phrase at one time or another.

I was diagnosed in February 1991, and quietly celebrated my five-year anniversary last year. Now another year has passed; I am cancer free and I am still a survivor. And this book is finished. In the weeks shortly after I was diagnosed, you could never have convinced me I would see this day. What a trip!

I'm reminded of a quote from the television show *Law and Order,* in which the character of the female police lieutenant says, "There are two kinds of women today—those who have breast cancer and those who are afraid of getting it." Unfortunately, breast cancer has touched nearly every woman's life in some way. You can talk to almost any woman and find that either she has had breast cancer or her sister has or her mother has or her daughter has or a friend has or a friend of her sister, mother, or daughter has. It affects us all. There are indeed two kinds of women, and both kinds know someone who has breast cancer.

When I was first diagnosed, I didn't know that there were only two kinds of women. I was frightened. I was devastated, and I felt completely alone. This doesn't mean that my husband wasn't there for me; he was. He was caring, loving, supportive, and honest. I had good, caring doctors, and I had many friends who were concerned about me and for me, but I still felt an isolating chill of fear and dread. When someone would say, "Well, we're all going to die someday," I wanted to retort, "But you don't have the threat of a recurrence." Unless you've had someone look you in the eye and tell you that you have cancer, you can't know how it feels.

Early during my "trip," or journey, as I have started thinking of it now, I spent a great deal of time combing the shelves in the local bookstores. I was searching for anything that would tell me how other women who had been told they had breast cancer felt and reacted and dealt with this disease. I wanted to hear how other women coped with all that goes along with having this disease. Would I ever be able to reclaim my former self, the person I was before breast cancer? Could I even hope sometime in the future to be able to go for a full day without the thought of having breast cancer being uppermost in my mind? I didn't particularly want books on recovery, prayer, the devotional life, or even stories from other survivors of cancers other than breast cancer.

After an initial, frantic binge, I no longer wanted more medical information or survival statistics. I didn't want to hear from women who had had breast cancer twenty years ago—except to hear they had survived. I wanted to know the stories of women who had just gone through or were currently experiencing what I was experiencing—dealing with the current treatments and the decisions necessarily arising from these treatments. I wanted and needed the company of women who spoke the same language because they were on the same journey.

I attended a support group briefly but found the focus of the group was reconstructive surgery. I think the words that helped me the most at that critical time, during that first year, were the words of encouragement my surgeon would offer. She was candid and direct, but when I was particularly anxious, she would offer me something positive. I know now that her use of examples from the stories of some of her other patients was especially meaningful for me—stories of real women who had breast cancer and were not only alive but were leading healthy and happy lives. Dr. Jeanne Ballinger, the woman who delivered to me the worst news of my life, helped me begin to believe that there is life after breast cancer.

During my own journey—this trip from diagnosis to surgery to chemo to today, with stops at grief, anxiety, fear, anger, loneliness, and hope—I have personally met many remarkable survivors, and I have recorded their stories. It is true that the stories in this book are stories of remarkable healing and determination and growth. But they are stories of humor and new ways of living and of the everydayness of getting on with life.

I have met many of these wonderful women in person, and some friends I have met on the Internet. There are some things that many of these women have in common, things that are highlighted or emphasized because of their breast cancer. Being told you have a chronic, life-threatening disease calls on you to find courage you didn't know you had. And frequently you find humor and honesty and a willingness to make yourself vulnerable to others who are facing the same disease and some of the same challenges.

This book is not for every woman who is living with breast cancer. Each woman's reaction to diagnosis and treatment is uniquely her own. But I do know many women want to hear other women's stories, just as I wanted to and still do. Interviewing and recording the stories from the women in this book has been an enriching and often hilarious experience.

I believe in the power of one woman's story to help another find pathways to her own healing. The personal stories I have assembled here reflect the courage and insight of some very ordinary but extraordinary women. I hope these stories will help women on their journeys know that they are not alone. They are members of a club none of us would choose to belong to; but this club, this sisterhood of survivors, has great wealth of knowledge, grace, wisdom, and joy. I am grateful to each woman here for giving me the gift of her experience to pass on to other women.

Charla Andson Honea

"Why are you worried about losing your breast? Your life is what you should be worried about." I overheard this comment in a doctor's office. Apparently the daughter was trying to help her mother adjust to her upcoming surgery.

This really pushed my button. Such a statement completely overlooks what might be a very important issue in a woman's life.

Yes, my life is more important than my breast. It is more important than my arm, my eyes, my hearing, even my job or my marriage. But a breast is more than a breast. It is a symbol of sex, our sex in particular. It is also a nurturing symbol. For many, the loss of a breast brings hurt, fear, and sorrow. To discount that fear or sorrow is insensitive and cruel.

I remember someone saying to me, "You'll never miss it."

Well, that person might not, but I do and so does my husband.

Each woman mourns the loss of a breast in a different way. Some deny the grief altogether. Some don't deal with it until things have "settled down" and they find they are expected to lead "normal lives," only they don't feel very normal. Some never experience acute grief over the loss. But what is important is that we respect each other enough to let each woman deal with her decision and her doctor's decision in her own way and in her own time. To ignore her feelings by telling her it doesn't matter robs her of her individuality.

When I first had my diagnosis and surgery, I wanted to get rid of that breast! My life was all I cared about. Now I feel its loss keenly and am considering reconstructive surgery, something I said at first I would never do. Life changes us in ways we may never expect.

I hope that that mother in the doctor's office was able to do what most breast cancer survivors must learn—to listen kindly to those who try to help but only cause pain, and to make her own decisions in consultation with her doctors.

Jan

Consider how you have reacted when someone has been insensitive to your feelings—before your diagnosis, during treatment, and now. Have your responses been different? If so, how?

When you've been through treatment, or are going through it, you need all the support and acknowledgment you can get. Often this will come from people you didn't know even cared, while the people you think care the most may not be there for you.

Some people are unable to get beyond their own fears—fear of *cancer*, of *death*, of *pain*. These fears can be so overwhelming that the only way for these people to deal with your illness is to run away from it. I have decided that I want to try to have patience with these people.

Right now my job is to fight the cancer, to hold onto life! I will accept the love and caring from wherever it comes. But I know my own inner strength will make the biggest difference.

I'm a two-and-a-half-year survivor. You just "gotta keep truckin' and take life as it comes." Life is too short even *without* cancer, but cancer does make it even more important to be your own self.

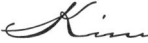

How have you responded to those people who have disappointed you?

I was fifty-two years old when I was diagnosed with breast cancer. I immediately thought about all the things I wanted to do before I die. Then I went out and bought rollerblades!

Four years later, I have had shoulder surgery for a rollerblading accident, changed professions, and am trying to deal with going in and out of remission. Life goes on!

Jannie

In what areas of your life do you experience spontaneity?

When I went to buy my "stick-on" prostheses (I had a bilateral mastectomy), the technician said, "You know we have some artificial nipples, don't you?" Well, maybe it was the way she phrased the question, but I just started laughing.

My immediate thought was, *Artificial nipples? More than two?* Oh, I could get several and put them in unexpected places. And not only that, I could wear two of them on each falsie. I could put one on my forehead and wait to see how long it would take someone to notice it. I could stick one on my cheek and tell my husband it is the new style now.

I was grateful for these lighthearted moments.

Agatha

What "lighthearted moments" do you especially recall during your journey since your diagnosis?

Many breast cancer survivors say their fear lessens as the years go by, but I find I still get scared sometimes. After ten years and good reports, I always get a little anxious when I go in for my annual checkup, or a new ache or pain comes along. "Wait a week," my oncologist says, "and then call." This advice has helped me more than once.

In my support group we always say, "Good luck and stay positive," but we also discuss how each of us needs to have a "pity party" once in a while. But such moods and needs do become less and less frequent.

No, I don't think you ever get over *all* the fear any more than you ever get over all other kinds of fears that have nothing to do with cancer. Sometimes my fear is very present to me during my day and sometimes it is totally forgotten. Yes, you do get to the point where breast cancer is not the first thing you think about when you wake up in the morning, but that may take a while.

When I was first diagnosed, I felt my life had been permanently changed for the worse and that I would live out the rest of my days with a cloud of worry and depression hanging over my head. Not true! I have sorted through so many things and resolved some significant life issues. I can honestly say I am happier now than I have ever been in my life—even before the breast cancer.

Lee

How have you grown more confident during your experience with breast cancer?

It is hard to know what to expect from chemotherapy because it varies from individual to individual. The side effects of chemo depend on the type of chemo the person is having. I had mine (CMF) on Friday afternoons, was sick Saturday, felt icky on Sunday, and was back to work on Monday. I lost no hair and was, all in all, very fortunate. It is my understanding that CAF causes stronger reactions.

The chemo did affect my teeth, but I had inferior teeth to begin with. I was due for an eye exam while I was having treatments, and the ophthalmologist suggested I wait until six months after completing treatments before getting new glasses because chemo can temporarily affect your eyes.

It would be easier, I think, if there were only one type of reaction to meds and then we would all know what to expect, but unfortunately, each of us is different. Weight gain is another variable. Some people lose a lot and some gain a lot and some experience no change. Makes no sense.

One thing is certain in all this. We need the support of our families and of each other. Sharing our experiences is one of the best gifts we can give others with breast cancer.

Peggy

Have you been able to support other women who are going through some of the same things you are experiencing?

I am currently undergoing chemo-
therapy and radiation therapy. My mother died of breast cancer
with metastasis to the bone. I started writing "letters" to her when
I was first diagnosed. This process has helped me work through
some things about my illness and fear as well as my relationship
with her. Here is one of the letters I wrote early on:

Dear Mom,

The breast cancer I feared all these years has happened to me.
When I thought I might get cancer someday, I assumed if it happened it would be when I was old. I remember that when you had
your mastectomy I thought of you as being "old." Now I am forty-
one, the same age as when you had your surgery, and it doesn't feel
old at all—in fact, it feels awfully young.

Weren't you scared, Mom? You must have been afraid, but I
didn't see that. I wish you had told me more about how you were
feeling. Maybe you wanted to, but you knew I wasn't ready to listen. I was scared, too.

When I was young and someone would tell me I had your smile
or your gestures, I was always surprised that there was something
in me of you that others could see. But as I grew older, I discovered
I was interested in the same things you were interested in. I went
into teaching, not to be like you but because that is who I am, too.

Now breast cancer is one more thing we have in commo\

I don't die from it. My doctor says I won't, because they c\

early and there are treatments available now that didn't exist when

you were diagnosed twenty years ago.

I wish you had not been taken from us when you were. I wish

we could be together and you could tell me how you dealt with

your fears so well.

Love,

Jan

Try writing a letter to someone you love and admire, living or dead.

My hair came out in clumps. It was short, and once it started coming out, I pulled out a lot of it.

I discovered several new hair products that got me through a hot summer. There are halo wigs. They give you the Friar Tuck look with bangs and hair over your ears and neck. Pop on a hat or scarf and you are ready to go. I found that an easier way to go for much of the summer.

I also bought some curly bangs. I would just tuck them in under my turban or hat and go! Another cool alternative.

I made up my mind to have as much fun with my hair loss as I could manage. For cooler weather I bought a long wig with curls. My own hair would never curl like this wig. I also have had a short wig that is closer to my original haircut.

I did discover some advantages to my hair loss. I didn't have to shave my legs or armpits. However, now that I am on a different chemo, my hair is growing back, and I seem to be shaving all the time!

The hair I missed the most was the hair in my nose. Because of my allergies I always had to keep tissues handy since there was nothing to stop the allergic reaction! I also lost my eyelashes and felt like I always had something in my eyes. I almost lost my eyebrows, but not quite.

I recommend the "Look Good, Feel Better" sessions offered by the American Cancer Society. I learned a lot about wigs and drawing eyebrows and stuff. I almost didn't go, but was glad I did; it was an uplifting experience.

Mary

What are some of the creative, even funny ways you have dealt with your appearance during your treatment?

I am a three-year breast cancer survivor. Once the initial shock of my diagnosis was over, I found that my general attitude seemed to have changed.

Before cancer, I was demure and quiet. Now I feel life is too short to put up with some things that I tolerated in the past. For instance, if someone is hollering at their dog or their child or swearing because they must wait in line, I'll say something to them and ask them to consider their actions and the feelings of others. There are a lot of things I wish I had done in the past. Well, I've been given a second chance and I'm going to use it!

Lou

In what ways has your attitude changed during your experience with breast cancer?

After I was diagnosed and had begun treatment, I tried to concentrate all my energy on getting better (what little energy I had). For me this meant making some major decisions about how I was living my life and being willing to let go of some things that before I got sick were very important to my self-image.

I started by leaving a well-paying but very stressful job and taking a less intense position. I began walking two to three miles five days a week. Then I planned a strategy for trying eventually to fulfill my dream of leaving the city and getting a home in the country. Just last month I found a little log house in the woods that I could afford and am now in the process of purchasing it.

Cancer made me realize how precious my life is and how short it can be. Even though I don't know what the future holds for me, I can certainly try to enjoy the present as much as possible and do those things that are healthful for me in body, mind, and spirit.

Alice

What are your dreams for your future? What steps can you take right now to begin making them a reality?

We survivors, who have been through the mill, must keep yelling "second opinion." Women with breast cancer shouldn't rely solely on the opinion of *one* doctor from *one* area of specialization for treatment of this disease. Some doctors tend to focus primarily on their own area for the treatment of breast cancer. As some people who are a little bitter say, a surgeon wants to "slash," a radiation oncologist wants to "burn," and a regular oncologist wants to "poison."

Sometimes surgery, radiation therapy, and chemotherapy may *all* be appropriate, sometimes only one or two. Each of us needs to get as much information as we can to make wise decisions that are right for us and that we can feel comfortable with.

Lee

What combination of treatments did you and your doctors decide on? To some people, the treatments for breast cancer may seem barbaric. Have you been able to see the treatment process as positive?

I have no family history of breast cancer. I was thirty-four years old when diagnosed. At that time I had a lumpectomy and was told by the surgeon that I would only have to have radiation, no chemotherapy.

When I went to the oncologist, he said I needed six months of chemotherapy. My lymph nodes were not involved, but I am glad I went to the oncologist and that I did what he recommended.

Because of my fibrocystic disease, in consultation with the oncologist I have now decided to have a double mastectomy with breast reconstruction. I prefer not have to continue to watch my breasts like a hawk!

If I had known all my tumor factors at the time of my original surgery, I probably would have had a double mastectomy then. But of course I'm not sure I would have. We can only deal with today's decisions today. Tomorrow's decisions must wait for tomorrow.

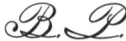

Sometimes we want to revise our decisions in light of new discoveries or new insight. What have been the most important factors to you in the decisions you have made? Why?

I am a six-year breast cancer survivor. Yes, it is possible to have a life after breast cancer and to think of a future and to deal with things other than cancer. For a while, it is hard to think of anything else. That is normal, we all go through that.

My support group has been a great help for me. It really helps to be able to relate to those who have experienced the same thoughts and feelings I am going through.

Another plus is that I have found people who really care about me, and I have made many friends. I get to meet people who have traveled the cancer journey. Some are still fighting the cancer, others are in remission, others are just now going on chemo.

It gives me strength to see these women going through this experience with courage, and it gives me the opportunity to give back to others. These survivors have taught me to look at the positive side.

I suppose that no matter what the circumstances are, there is always some positive aspect to any situation. For me, breast cancer has provided a good kick in the rear to get me started rethinking my life and finding out just what my priorities should be.

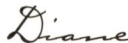

Do your friends and associates try to help you see "the positive side"?

When I had my HDC/SCR (high-dose chemotherapy/stem cell recovery), I would go in and be put on a machine that would take my blood from my body. Then the doctors would take the stem cells out of my blood and return the rest of the blood to my body. This procedure would take up to five days, because they had to make sure that they got enough of the stem cells.

I had to lie there a long time, and as they would take the stem cells out of my blood, at some points my body would begin to shake. If this happened the nurse would feed me Tums or calcium pills. She said the process tends to cause hypocalcemia.

After a few days, they had gotten enough cells and I just needed to have some scans and a lung test done to make sure I was strong enough for this procedure.

On December 7, 1995, I was admitted to the hospital. That night around 11:00 P.M. they started the high-dose chemo. I was hoping I wouldn't have to have it until the next day, but no such luck. I had chemo around the clock for three days. Then I had three days of rest. After that they injected the stem cells back into my body. Then I had to wait for my blood count to come back up. The chemo made me very sick—sicker than I have ever been. Mostly I just slept.

Then on December 28, 1995, my count had come up enough that I got to go home. I was still very sick, and wasn't eating. I couldn't stand any food smells and only wanted to sleep. But it was a lot easier to be at home.

I knew I was beginning to recover. It was a long time before I really started to feel like, "Hey, I'm alive and I kind of like it again. Maybe I will enjoy some of the things I did before."

I remember reading an article when I was first diagnosed about a woman whose cancer had returned. I thought to myself, *Well, I hope this cancer never comes back because I don't think I could handle it!* But I have handled it—four times now.

I am still alive after ten years and for that I am thankful. In the beginning of this disease, I didn't want to admit that I had anything really serious. For me, denial was the best way to go. I figured I would just do what the doctor said and get on with my life. Now I can deal with my cancer and actively fight it. I refuse to sit around and mope. I decided to have all these procedures done because *I want to live.*

Deborah

Have you found you can do things you never dreamed you would be capable of doing? Who has helped you the most in being able to get through those difficult times?

I went for both breasts at the same time—a bilateral mastectomy. I had lobular carcinoma, less than one and a half centimeters, and my doctor wanted to do a lumpectomy with radiation. I insisted on a bilateral mastectomy. My husband (a pathologist) was the only one who agreed with me. That was four years ago, and I have never regretted my decision. The breast with the tumor had atypical hyperplasia in every lobule. My other breast was completely healthy with no abnormal pathology. I had reconstruction this summer and now have a matched set, although I went flat for four years. The only time I wore any form at all was with a bathing suit.

But this was *my personal choice*. This decision was right for me. It might not be the right decision for anyone else. We really need to pay attention to our gut feelings as well as our heads when making these tough decisions. And we need to take our time.

Jellie

On what do you tend to rely in making important decisions—intuition or logic? If both, where does your confidence lie—in intuition or in the rational?

I believe that waiting to hear whether you have breast cancer is the worst part of it all. I can well remember the time between my mammogram and biopsy. After I knew for sure, one way or the other, I could begin to deal with it.

I was forty-three when I was diagnosed. I had lost my father about a month before my diagnosis, and I lost my mother about six months after treatment. It seems like these things come in bunches. But I keep telling myself to hang in there. And I find that I feel pretty good about things now.

Laurie

How are you and your family handling your illness along with the other stresses that are present in your lives?

Since my diagnosis and treatment, I have to say overall that I have more good or tolerable days than bad days, and I want to be sure to savor them. Here are some things I've enjoyed lately.

Watching a pheasant pecking at scattered birdseed under the feeder hanging from the tree in our backyard. Seeing him hiding behind the bushes when children walk by on the street and then darting out to eat some more.

Seeing a fat, bushy gray squirrel figuring out how to get at the same feeder. He solved the problem by running out along the branch holding the feeder and then dropping onto it from above. Way to go, squirrel! Have all the seed you want.

Being awakened in the middle of the night by our dog's barking and finding that he was barking at a doe and her two fawns in our backyard. They didn't care about the dog. They were busy scrounging seed from another bird feeder near the house and munching on my peony bush. I'm toying with the idea of putting out hay for them, but I don't want to support a whole herd of deer.

Waking up and finding that my orange tabby cat has curled up next to my shoulder and is washing my face as though she is "mom cat" and I am her kitten.

Watching my granddaughters decorate the Christmas tree. They felt important to be responsible for this crucial activity. We can always do some surreptitious rearrangement later.

E.R.

What simple pleasures have you experienced in the past week?

"Nerves" are a common problem during and after the initial treatment phase of breast cancer. I started having panic attacks several years after I finished chemotherapy treatments. It is my understanding that chemo affects all of your body, including your brain.

Fortunately, I now take Xanax and Prozac and feel great. Sometimes we try so hard to be strong and brave during the treatments. I think after they are completed and we start to relax, the mental stuff kicks in. Cancer is terrifying and it is, I think, to be expected that some of us will have a problem with our nerves afterwards. It is nothing to be ashamed of, and we should not think we have failed when we must ask for help with our feelings.

Peggy

Have you given yourself permission to acknowledge you have some anxiety or "blues" and to ask for help for your emotional well-being?

Breast cancer can affect anyone close to us in a variety of ways. When I was diagnosed, things really started going downhill with my husband. We got counseling, and after eighteen months things are finally taking a turn for the better. It seems my husband was terrified that I would "leave" him because of my illness—that I would die or that I would change so much that I might leave home.

I found some real true-blue friends while I was going through my treatments. I found that my pain eased as I met and made new friends.

Not only have I been changed by this experience, but those close to me have been changed as well.

Betsy

Have you explored how your illness might be affecting those closest to you in unexpected ways?

My first surgery was a lumpectomy followed by radiation, but some of the cancer cells were just as stubborn as I am, and the radiation must not have gotten them all. All my lymph nodes were clean then.

One year later I found another lump and underwent an MRM and chemo. The day I was getting ready to go home after that second surgery, the nurse brought me a gift the hospital usually gives to mastectomy patients, a very pretty, soft camisole with pockets for two falsies. This gift was designed for the patient to use until she could get her own prosthesis.

I asked the nurse how to "assemble this ensemble." I am small-busted, and I lost only my right breast to cancer. After we put in the one falsie, she looked at me and I looked at her, and then we both burst out laughing together. Needless to say, my new right "breast" was about twice the size of the left one! I found out later that you pull the stuffing out of the falsie until you get it down to the right size.

It hasn't been easy surviving breast cancer by any means, but I've never lost my sense of humor. Thank God for that! I'm doing fine now, am on tamoxifen, and am looking forward to the day when I become a full-fledged doctor.

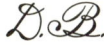

How well have you done at keeping your sense of humor during your diagnosis and treatment?

I guess I see this whole breast cancer experience as just that—an experience. One of life's experiences that God (or whoever is in charge!) has sent my way to let me learn firsthand some things I needed to know. "Why?" is not a burning question with me, because to "Why?" I would say "Why not?"

I'm not totally accepting of this "experience." I have days when I rant and rave and am really *pissed* about the whole thing! But I also see it as an opportunity to learn about myself and about this disease. And I have met so many fascinating people throughout this experience. For me breast cancer has really been a gift in some ways.

One thing I have learned is that I don't think I'll ever be truly "cured" mentally. My mind always says "What if ..." whenever something new shows up—whether it's an abnormal test result, a new ache or pain, or just something that feels different. I am cautious but optimistic.

Lately, though, I've come to wonder whether others around me are *too* cautious. I feel as though my family doctor doesn't see me as myself anymore but only as his "breast cancer patient." Consequently, every little abnormality of mine seems to cause him to panic. I wonder sometimes whether "WARNING: BREAST CANCER PATIENT!" is written in big, bold, red letters on my chart! Just because I have (had) breast cancer does not mean that the disease is my primary way of thinking of myself, nor should it be the main identifier others apply to me. I am still a whole person and I resist bring treated like someone who has passed to the other side of some invisible barrier and is now among the "walking dead."

Gay

Sometimes it is difficult to appreciate the fact that our health care providers are vulnerable to the same kinds of insecurities we are. Have you experienced this? How did it make you feel?

I had a bilateral mastectomy and tram flap reconstruction eight months ago. I would do it again in a heartbeat. My plastic surgeon arranged for me to talk to one of her patients who had had a tram flap. This woman was so helpful; she even met me for lunch and showed me her new breasts! Maybe telling my experience will help others who are considering tram flap surgery.

My surgery took ten hours. Afterwards I felt as though I'd been hit by a Mack truck. I had a close friend who stayed in the hospital with me. You can't imagine how nice it was to open my eyes and see a loving face, someone to feed me ice chips and put a cool cloth on my forehead. If your hospital will allow this, I highly recommend that you do it.

I wanted no visitors, and my friends respected that wish. I'm glad I did that, since I'm the kind of person who feels that she must entertain guests! Getting out of bed the day after surgery was pretty scary, but the thought of it was much worse than the actual event. And it did get easier, just as they promised.

I had to wear circulation booties, and they drove me nuts. They feel a little like someone is grabbing your feet every few seconds.

Don't forget to bring Chapstick! I got off the morphine pump as soon as possible. It is great, but it wears off too fast. Percodan works much better. During breathing treatments, I coughed up a little blood, but that was from the tube inserted during the surgery.

The first two days are a little foggy, but improvement came by leaps and bounds after that. I went home on day seven and my friend came with me. She is an angel. I rented a hospital bed for a month, and I'm so glad I did. Lying flat was impossible. I put a plastic lawn chair in my shower. It is hard to stand up for a long time, and nothing feels better than to sit there and let the warm water run down your back.

Be sure you have nighties that button down the front. It's impossible to put things on over your head. Buy milk, juice, laundry soap, etc., in small containers because you aren't allowed to do very much lifting.

You will have to learn some new body mechanics. Sitting up from a lying-down position is hard, but if you turn on your side and push up with your arms, it's a lot easier. Some areas of my skin felt a little like a cross between having a bad sunburn and being rubbed by coarse sandpaper. This is normal. I had shooting pains that felt a little like sparks. It was the nerves coming back to life. I drove a car at five weeks. I could have done it sooner, but I didn't feel comfortable with it. It has now been eight months. I'm not back 100 percent, but pretty close. My breasts have healed nicely, with no complications. They are beautiful! And the tummy tuck is an added bonus.

Cynthia

Have you had reconstructive surgery? If not, what is your impression of what it would be like?

I had just spent two years on Weight Watchers and was almost to my goal when my breast cancer was diagnosed! Fortunately, I wasn't totally to my goal and still had enough abdominal tissue to do the tram flap!

Just goes to show you that no matter what you may plan for your life, fate sometimes steps in and changes your course. It is better to be able to "go with the flow" and make life the best you can even in a bad situation.

Sometimes my students complain that life isn't fair. I have to tell them that life is *not* fair and that's just the way it is! But that doesn't mean that you can't make the best of it!

Jan

In what ways can someone go about making life better whatever the circumstance?

I am forty-five years old. In December 1991 I was diagnosed with stage IV breast cancer. The cancer had already spread to my liver. My friends and family thought I was dying, and I did too. But my doctor insisted that I not give up. I had radiation treatment on the affected areas of the bone. I also had all sorts of chemotherapy. For two years I was very weak from the cancer and from the treatments, so sick that I stayed in bed almost all the time. But gradually I began to feel better.

Finally, my oncologist said I was strong enough and healthy enough to have a stem cell transplant. He told me it might help me or it might not. The decision was up to me.

I was terribly frightened, but decided to go ahead with the stem cell transplant. I decided I wanted to do everything I could to survive as long as I could. I tried so hard to be brave and to keep up my hopes. I had the procedure in November of 1995. My doctor is very kind. He always tries to tell me just what to expect, as much as he can.

I have not had to have chemotherapy at all since the transplant. I know full well that stage IV breast cancer is life-threatening, and some people act like it's a death sentence. But I feel I have been given a second chance for happiness for another four years or so, maybe even ten. God is with me, and God and my doctors saved my life, at least for the time being.

I have learned *never* to give up, regardless of the odds.

Laura

Where does your hope lie? In science or in your faith, or both?

I had a mastectomy with reconstruction in December 1993, and I wouldn't have done it any other way. It was devastating enough to find out I had cancer without having to adjust to an "empty" chest.

When I regained consciousness after surgery, it was so wonderful to look down and see a "breast" there and not a "hole." And I have never had to worry about a prosthesis falling out.

I felt that since I had to recover from the mastectomy surgery itself anyway, why not have reconstruction at the same time so that all healing can take place at one time? Besides, after three kids, it was nice to have a flat abdomen again!

Part of the healing process is not only physical, but emotional, and having reconstruction definitely helped my emotional healing. It is wonderful to be able to wear regular bras and not have to worry about special mastectomy bras.

I am in a support group called "Image Reborn," which includes mostly women who have had or are contemplating having breast reconstruction after mastectomy. It is a wonderful, positive group and has been a great morale booster. For me, and I can only speak for myself, reconstruction is definitely worth it!

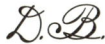

Each of us has to make her own decision about reconstruction. What are/were your priorities when you have considered this for yourself?

I had an MRM by choice. At age 61, I care very little about the missing breast. But I *insist* on each woman's right to choose between options—to mourn a poor choice, if that happens, to mourn the loss of the breast(s) if she chooses, and to mourn any darn thing she wants. Mourning can be healthy, and it gets us through the hard moments toward an equally healthy acceptance of what is and must be.

Nancy J.

Is there an area in your life of unresolved internal conflict? Is there an area where you think you might want to do some "healthy mourning"?

It is heartbreaking when breast cancer recurs or metastasizes. But the surprising thing is that once it happens—well, it's not really as bad as we feared! Does that make sense?

Somehow God grants us the strength to do what we must to survive and go on surviving no matter what! My first diagnosis and lumpectomy was ten years ago. I also had radiation. The mastectomy on the second breast was in February 1992 and was followed by six months of CAF and four years of tamoxifen. Then this past winter I was sick a lot with bronchitis and pneumonia, only to discover in May that I had breast cancer metastasis to my left lung and maybe a rib.

I stopped tamoxifen, began Arimidex, and really began to feel quite hopeless! Although I was going through the motions of doing the right things, I was paralyzed by the idea that there is no cure for advanced breast cancer! Somehow I couldn't get my mind to accept a cure or lengthy remission for me—only for others!

The Arimidex didn't help. In fact, we know that the disease has progressed because it is now in both of my lungs, my chest, my lymph nodes, the bone of my right upper arm, a rib, and a few scattered possibles in other bones. Now I have switched to Taxol.

I am finally encouraged and am beginning to have some hope for a remission. My last CT scan showed a reduction both in lungs and chest lymph nodes and no breast cancer in the liver at all! If I can't be cured of breast cancer, maybe I can at least learn to live with it just as others have learned to live with incurable diseases such as diabetes and MS. I plan to continue taking my meds and my treatments and maintaining a fairly high quality of life for as long as I can.

Whether you are young or old, breast cancer is not a death sentence.

Nan

What is the worst thing that could happen in your life? How do you think you would cope?

Even though my kids come home for Christmas (two or three days), I find myself crying occasionally when unpacking special ornaments—my grandmom's or mom's or something the kids made.

But I think this reaction is part of a good thing—good times and good memories. I have started writing down the history of each particular keepsake and ornament (just in case the kids forget where we got it or who made it). I plan to make three copies when the list is complete, one for each of my children. This is the second year for the list and I hope to finish it soon.

God gave us memory to help us keep alive in our hearts those people we have cared about the most. Writing down funny or memorable comments/events can be passed down, too. It does help.

Millie

In what ways do you honor or keep in your heart those whom you love who have preceded you in death?

I went back to my plastic surgeon yesterday, and he thinks that a portion of the flap from my tram flap reconstructive surgery has "failed" and that I'm not healing properly. He says I don't have adequate circulation for the flap and so my recovery will be very slow.

He's going to be pretty busy in that follow-up surgery getting rid of scar tissue and making the nipples. In the meantime, he says, there's nothing I can do but continue to take good care of the wound (daily cleaning, antibiotic ointment, dressings) and that it will eventually heal, but slowly. He won't/can't give an estimate of time, but he made it clear that at the least we're talking about weeks. He says he gets about one case a year that simply doesn't heal quickly.

I'm really sick of this! I cry every morning when I have to change the dressings and spread on the antibiotic ointment. I've started to use sanitary napkins over my initial dressing because I'm sick of bleeding all over my bras and shirts.

But I've decided I can't continue to dwell on all this, and I need to get on with my life. So I'll just deal with my breast each day after my shower and then try to forget about it. I hesitated a little about talking about this with others because I know sometimes it is frightening to hear about things that can go wrong. But my case is clearly the exception. I'm convinced I will get better with time, and that will make everything worth it.

Elaine

If you have had breast cancer surgery, how do you feel about the changes that have occurred? How do you picture yourself two years from now? Five years?

I was diagnosed with breast cancer two and a half years ago and had surgery and chemo. A friend of mine, who is single, has recently had a mastectomy and is undergoing chemotherapy. She has never asked for my help on anything during the time since her diagnosis. But last week she told me three times when her upcoming appointments for her treatments are.

It occurred to me that she might be trying to tell me she would like someone to go with her to her appointments. If she has a hard time asking for or receiving help, she may not be able to articulate her need. I called her and told her I would like to take her to her appointments. She seemed quite pleased although she did not say very much.

I took her for her second treatment last week, and at lunch afterward she started to share some of her feelings about what is happening to her. Tears came to her eyes as she described her mother's death from breast cancer. When I started to make a suggestion she said, "I don't want to bother you, and I am not asking you to solve my problems. I just need someone to talk to who understands."

I must respect her privacy, but I can still support her. Open, honest, and caring communication—just listening and talking about feelings without offering solutions, suggestions, or advice—may be difficult but is often very powerful.

Lee

Do you have someone who will just listen to you and not try to control or advise? Is there someone for whom you could be such a friend?

Dear Mom,

I am so scared of having the mastectomy and chemotherapy. A woman called me the other day. She has been through her own breast cancer diagnosis and treatment. She heard about me through a mutual friend, and she came over to talk with me and to try to ease my fears about this surgery. It was so wonderful to see her and to see how good she looks! I feel much better about it now.

I remember when you were in the hospital in such pain after your cancer had metastasized to your bones. A bouncy little woman named Marty came to visit you. She had a colorful scarf around her head in a turban and she looked so good! You called her your "angel," because she came to you, understood what you were going through, and gave you hope. I didn't understand how important a person like that could be at the time, but now I have had my own angel come, in the person of Pam.

I have begun to understand what an angel really is. One of God's messengers, an angel goes before us and shows us the way, always saying, "Don't be afraid." Now I know that God will be with me, no matter what comes. I'm glad that you had your angel, too.

Love,

Jan

Has anyone helped you in unexpected ways? Do you feel that someday you might be able to help other women the way Pam helped Jan?

I have breast cancer that has metastasized to the bone, and I am still undergoing chemo treatments every three weeks. I have had breast cancer for eight years, seven years in remission. Then in September 1995, my breast cancer recurred in the bones. I will receive my eighteenth round of chemo tomorrow.

The good news is that I have great doctors and a faith that is unshakable. I know that miracles of healing happen, but I realize that most of the time they don't. We don't understand always, but I believe God always has a higher purpose or plan to carry out through our lives. I feel God has been healing me gradually since my breast cancer recurred. I continue to get outstanding reports from my doctor.

I pray for courage to face each day. God helps protect me from fear, anxiety, and the unknown. I try to trust and rely on God's strength. I know my life is in God's hands.

Lil

What or who provides you with spiritual sustenance during life's rough times?

The other night I got home and started to undress to take a bath. To my dismay I discovered that my prosthesis was not in my bra. I couldn't even remember whether I had put it in when I dressed that morning. Hurriedly I put on my bathrobe and started looking for it around the house—in the bedroom and in both bathrooms.

As I went through the living room, my thirteen-year-old daughter asked me what was wrong. "I can't find my booby," I told her and wandered back to the bedroom. Finally I found it under a pile of clothes. Boy, was I relieved! I kept having visions of it having fallen out somewhere during the day and laughing about what people would make of it when they found it.

Later I went back to the living room with it in my hand and told my daughter that I had found it. She had never really looked at it closely before. I showed it to her and told her it was kind of like a beanbag. I asked her whether she would like to play catch. You should have seen the dirty look I got.

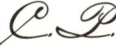

How do you feel about trying to put others at ease about your illness by using a bit of humor?

Hope. I have been thinking about the notion of hope. We all have two choices, one is to hope, the other is *not* to hope. Until I know for myself that my body has grown tired and I need to leave this world, I will hope.

When I was only fourteen years old, I had a terrible disease and my parents were told I had only three months to live. I was very ill. What if my parents had believed the so-called experts?

Hope is a decision. It is a decision each of us has to make for ourselves—"a faith thing." "No hope," according to Webster, implies "no expectation of success." Well, this certainly doesn't apply to me!

Angela

What is the single most important thing that keeps you hopeful or optimistic?

The entire time I was on chemo I was counting the days until I would be finished—no more treatments—and feel free. Also, during that time, I was upbeat, enthusiastic, and optimistic. I felt I was in good hands medically and that the doctors and I were actively doing everything we could to effect a possible cure.

Well, finally the treatments were over and I started on tamoxifen. Instead of being jubilant and happy, as I had expected to be, I became anxious and sad, for the first time really since my diagnosis and surgery. Slowly I began to despair and feel very vulnerable. I became anxious thinking the cancer could move back in on me and "take over."

I realized that while I had been on chemo I felt safe and protected for at least those few months. Suddenly I had to "go it alone."

I asked my doctor whether the tamoxifen, which was blocking the estrogen's effects throughout my body, could be affecting my emotions. He said this occurs with some women on tamoxifen.

Then I started worrying about whether my anxiety could make me more vulnerable to the cancer—I started worrying about worrying. Finally I thought, *This is stupid. You need to get help to feel better.*

I did get help—medication and counseling. I feel fine now, but this totally unexpected turn for me taught me we cannot really predict anything. So I started intentionally to try to relax and to take things as they come.

Louise

Since none of us can truly know what the future holds, in what ways do you try to focus on living today rather than trying to anticipate what tomorrow might bring?

When they told me I had cancer, I vomited, right there in front of the doctor. I have never had anything jolt me like that news. I was terrified. I just knew I would be dead soon!

But I have really surprised myself. I have completed my treatments and as time goes on I feel a little better each day. I never thought I would, but I do.

I have prayed and prayed and prayed; I have never prayed so much in my life. Prayer has helped me more than anything else in dealing with my reaction to having this disease.

Penelope

Have you participated in meditation or prayer? If so, how do you feel it has helped you?

Sometimes while I was on CMF chemo, I worried that it might be causing brain damage. One day I was talking to a friend about setting up a lunch date and was looking at the calendar. I couldn't figure out what day it was, let alone what day Tuesday the following week would be. I felt like I'd really *lost* it! It was scary! But I have learned through talking to others that this is not uncommon. This kind of disorientation subsides after chemotherapy is over. I have always been sort of an airhead and now I try to blame it on the chemo, but I write myself a lot of notes, just as I did before chemo.

Gail

As you have moved into your experience with breast cancer, what unexpected occurrences have been frightening to you? How have you handled them?

My breast cancer was diagnosed in October 1994. Had a biopsy/lumpectomy procedure. In December 1994 I had a mastectomy with immediate reconstruction. I started chemo in January 1995. The doctors removed twenty lymph nodes, and eleven were positive. They also discovered several other cancerous spots in my breast that had not shown up on the mammogram.

When I saw the oncologist, I was told that my cancer was considered to be a stage III. At the time I was only thirty-five years old and raising two kids by myself. The oncologist started telling me about stem cell transplant. I researched it and asked lots of questions.

After much thought, I agreed with the doctor that this was the best choice for me. I had the actual transplant done in May 1995, right after my birthday. I spent a lot of time throwing up and sleeping (can't throw up when sleeping, so that's how I solved that little problem). As of now, I am still cancer free.

For me, this decision was the right one. Do I still worry about getting sick again? Sure I do, but for the time being I am okay. I'm relatively healthy now, raising my kids and working.

I had a lot of help, though. My family and friends were great. The hospital stay was about three weeks. Different people came over every night to take care of my kids so they could stay in our home. And after the hospital stay, I ended up having home nursing care for another two to three weeks. After that, I also did five weeks of radiation. But, as I said, at the moment everything is very encouraging for me.

Debbie

What have you been able to do in your life that you would never have predicted you would be able to do?

I have a close friend who has been "smothering" me since my surgery. She tells me she thinks about me every day. I have tried to tell her I am fine, and breast cancer is not the only subject I want to discuss. I think she means well, but my life does involve lots of things other than this disease. She has lost a few friends to cancer, and this may be the reason she is acting this way.

I discussed this with my counselor. She suggested that my friend might think she is going to lose me and she is also getting "hit in the face" with her own mortality. The counselor said some people treated her own husband this way when he had prostate cancer, while other people acted as though cancer is contagious and you can catch it just by talking about it!

One day last month my friend and I were having lunch together. I finally just told her, "Look, I'm the same person I've always been. I'm not going anywhere. I have a good prognosis, and I am ready to get on with living my life. Why don't we limit our discussions of health issues to once a week? Then the rest of the time we can relax and enjoy being together."

She seems better now and to have relaxed some. We laugh and talk together, and I am no longer concerned that my disease will end our friendship.

Andrea

Some people will always see you first as a cancer "victim" and then as a person. How are you handling these situations?

Dear Mom,

My friends always kid me about what a good husband I have. Len is truly a "nineties man." He is sensitive to my feelings, and he will hang in there and talk things through.

When I got back one day from seeing my plastic surgeon, I was kind of bummed out because he had to leave the drain in. I had really looked forward to having it out so that I could shower again! Thank heavens Len didn't try to answer my griping with anything but a hug and an "I know." Mother, how did you deal with your cancer? Did you ever have anyone say to your gripes and fears, "I know"?

Mom, I wish that I could tell you "I know," because I think I really do know, now. I know that I have been spared a lot of the disfigurement of a mastectomy because of my reconstruction, but when I look at my scars I still long for the body I had before. I know how hard it is to feel like having sex when you don't feel sexy. I was able to get some sexy nightgowns that cover the scars. This helps me, along with the good talks I have had with Len about how I feel.

Some people say, "It's only a breast. It's not like losing an arm or a leg." We try to make it seem less important, and I guess a breast is less important in the sense that losing it doesn't handicap you in any way, really. But my breasts have always, right or wrong, been very important to my sense of my own sexuality, and so the loss of one is hard. Our culture makes such a big deal of women's breasts. I've become especially conscious of that since my mastectomy. Seeing other women's breasts that don't have scars only reminds me that mine don't look that way anymore.

Mother, somehow you worked through these issues all on your own. I only wish I had been part of how you worked it out. I know it would help me now.

Love,

Jan

How important are your breasts to your sense of your sexuality? What measures are you taking to regain or enhance your sense of yourself as a sexual being?

I had a mastectomy in April 1995.

I was very fortunate. I had stage I, and no chemo or radiation. But I became really anxious when I started reading the breast cancer survival statistics. I read everything I could, and I was especially concerned because my docs think I have genetic breast cancer. I have sisters, cousins, aunts, and nieces who could be next.

While I was being so consumed with cancer survival stats, a lifelong friend was hit and killed by a seventeen-year-old drunk driver. That was a great lesson for me.

I still worry and wish I didn't, still read everything I can. But when I consider my situation rationally, I think there are just too many variables. I have one aunt who is twenty-one years out, another thirteen, and one aunt who died because she didn't see the doc when she found the lump. My mother-in-law lived six years after her mastectomy, but she could not have chemo because of so many other problems.

I believe God doesn't promise us length of life, only fullness of life if we embrace our faith, whatever that faith may be.

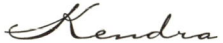

It is hard to live in the gray areas of our lives. Some of us yearn for guarantees where there are none. How do you cope with your major doubts or questions?

I have two lively cats. One of my first worries about having a saline implant in my reconstructive surgery was that one of these dear animals would wreak havoc with my implant.

You see, one of the cats, Alfred, seems to think people are walking trees. He always wants to be up on your shoulder. He loves being carried around, and he sometimes jumps up unexpectedly. I had horrible visions of spouting saline. Just one more reason for me to smile.

Millie

Do you have companion animals that make you smile? For many people they can be a delight and a source of comfort.

We have a wonderful sixteen-year-old daughter. When I was diagnosed with breast cancer, my husband sat her down and told her about it, letting her know that he would be there for both of us.

I wanted him to tell her because he is her stepfather of only two years, and I felt it was important they bond more now. It seems to have worked. After he told her, she went to her room for a few minutes and then came out and sat next to me on the couch, put her head on my shoulder, and let her tears flow. I rubbed her head and told her to let it out.

Although I am a very private person, I told her it was perfectly fine for her to tell whomever she wished. I felt it was important that she be able to speak openly with her friends and teachers. But I cautioned her ahead of time about other girls who might say hurtful things without meaning to, such as, "That means you're going to get it, too." This didn't happen often, thank goodness, but once or twice is enough.

Liz

How have you helped those closest to you to deal publicly with their having a "cancer patient" in the family?

I don't know the survival rates for women with breast cancer, because statistics really turn me off. But I do know about being scared! Fear can be especially difficult when you have a close family member or friend die of breast cancer while you're undergoing surgery and treatment.

I've been on this journey since my first diagnosis in December 1986, but I only recently discovered I'm now stage IV and that my cancer is incurable. That has been really hard to deal with, as well as my two- to five-year prognosis!

I am beginning to see that I've been paralyzed by statistics. I want to caution everyone with breast cancer to get your eyes off survival statistics and onto something else that will give you the hope and the inspiration you need to beat those odds!

I believe we all need to stay informed and do all we can to increase our life expectancy—in the areas of nutrition, physical exercise, and the spiritual life. I don't mean we ought to be ostriches with our heads in the sand, but we must not focus on a specific time span for our lives. Only God knows how much time each of us has, and trusting in God helps me deal with my fear.

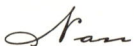

Have you found yourself focusing on survival statistics? If so, how have you gone about putting those statistics in the proper perspective?

Next Friday my plastic surgeon will put on my nipple. He could use a piece of skin from under my arm or a piece of skin from my inner thigh, but I said I wanted to go for the tattoo so the color would match the other side.

It has been one year since my reconstruction began. I have been told that the longer you wait, the more "in place" your breast will be.

The skin needs to stretch to where it will "hang" naturally. Otherwise, if the nipple or tattoo is put on too soon, it could end up pointing at your shoe or looking to the right or the left. I think three years is pretty safe, however. That boob has stretched to the max, no doubt.

T. J.

Do you become frustrated with waiting? What is the most important thing, person, or event you are waiting for now?

A diagnosis of breast cancer is *not* a death sentence. These days a lot can be done with surgery, radiation therapy, and chemotherapy. Most women are doing just fine, especially when the cancer is caught early. Also, most people go through chemo and radiation therapy without much difficulty. Yes, there are unpleasant side effects, and yes, I'd rather not have gone through it, but it is not necessarily the scary horror show most people think of.

Most of the women I know who have had chemo (including me) worked full-time. My advice to newly diagnosed women would be to try to relax. I know that sounds impossible. But at least try not to be overcome by panic and fear. And try to let some light and humor into what may at first seem to be a horrible experience.

Do you have a sport or hobby that helps you relax? Is it something you need to start doing again *now*?

She told me she knew that because of her breast cancer, the career she had planned on would never be. We were both sitting in the oncologist's office and had just started chatting.

"What career do you think will never be?" I asked. "A lot of women survive your stage of cancer." Then I remembered how I had bagged medical school because I thought I wouldn't live, even though the odds were all in my favor. "Life does go on and it is even more important now to live it like you want," I said. She nodded, seeming to consider this new perspective.

I happened to run into her two months later in a bookstore. After we greeted each other, she said, "You know, I thought a lot about what you said, and I have decided to go ahead and start law school this fall."

"Congratulations!" I patted her on the shoulder, "That's one for our side—*for* women and *against* letting breast cancer destroy our dreams."

Lila

Have you let go of any dreams that were important to before you were diagnosed? Would you like to reconsider them now?

I attend a support group for women who have recurrent breast cancer. One evening we decided to try to create the most unusual pinup calendar any of us had ever seen. We decided to put together a group calendar of all the major events in our experience with breast cancer. I went first and put a little hat on the calendar to represent the day I lost my hat and felt snow hitting my bald head. Lori put a little Kermit on the calendar because she always felt as though she looked green after her chemo treatments.

MaryAnn put the top to her swimsuit on the wall calendar because she vividly remembers a bright sunny day at the pool when she did a beautiful dive into the water. When she surfaced and looked around, she saw her prosthesis on top of the water, out of reach, floating away.

We had dozens of other pinups and stories. Before the evening was over, we were literally rolling on the floor laughing for about an hour! Great fun and great medicine!

J. J.

Have you had any humorous events in your breast cancer experience? What events or experiences have caused you to laugh lately?

Notwithstanding my breast cancer, I have always been the "Christmas Lady" wherever we've lived around the world. My mom, my sister, and I always made ornaments and sent them to each other. Something that has helped me is to divide the ornaments into four groups (one for each of our three kids and one for my husband and me).

I use those really neat paper boxes (you know, the ones that hold reams of copier paper for the office) with the lift-off tops. Little by little, I've given each "child" his or her special ornaments that Gramma made for them, as well as favorites from Germany (selfishly, I've kept the wooden ones for us—they'll get those someday).

Paring down the sizable number of ornaments has actually allowed me to have a nostalgic time in my mind with my mom, who passed away eight years ago. And readying those boxes for my kids (but not giving them to them yet) has allowed me to reduce my own collection to a more manageable size even though I still have too many.

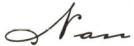

What activities might help you emotionally as well as help bring an enhanced sense of order to your life?

I know about the fear. I've never been cancer free since I was diagnosed in 1995. But I have a friend whom I love very much and she is cancer free after six years; however, each day she lives in fear that the cancer will return. She is beautiful, healthy, bright, and very active, but she still lives in fear.

There are no guarantees once you've fought and "won" the battle with breast cancer. I believe in continued prayer and always being hypervigilant regarding your body and how it feels and works. I try not to freak out with each little ache and pain but to be aware of any substantial changes and *not* be afraid to call my oncologist to discuss them.

Each of us is a survivor and a special person, whether or not she is in an active fight against this disease. We do need to be kind to ourselves and to each other.

Cindi

Do you feel as special now as you did before breast cancer? If yes, how? If no, why not?

When the doctor told me that I had to have my breast removed, the first thing I did when I got home was undress, look at myself in the mirror, get in the shower, and cry until I was so exhausted I couldn't cry anymore. Then I started trying to learn all I could about my disease.

The next thing I did was make love to my fiancé, but I waited until we went on vacation the next week to break the news to him. We were not engaged at that time. We got engaged *after* my surgery. We cried together and vowed to get through it together somehow.

Today I still cry at times, but together we're doing great. I can't wait to finish up chemo so we can get on with our lives and wedding plans.

Ronlene

What was the first thing you did after you learned your diagnosis? The second? The third?

Recently I was contacted by a woman whose seventy-two-year-old mother had just been diagnosed with breast cancer and was refusing the treatment recommended by her doctors, including chemo and radiation. The daughter had been given my name because I am a ten-year breast cancer survivor. I have tried to study this disease inside and out because right now I am no longer in remission.

I reminded her that her mother may just remember from her youth that anyone who had cancer died; anyone who had chemotherapy was really, really sick and then died anyway; and anyone who had radiation was also really, really sick and died!

Today things have changed. There are many new and better treatments and possibilities for cure. I suggested she have her mother read information from the American Cancer Society and talk to other breast cancer patients, especially those who are several years post op and who have a positive attitude. It could really change her outlook and her perspective!

We agreed that most of all she needed to be there for her mother in love and support—whatever her mother decides. It is her life and her body, after all!

Nan

Ignorance feeds fear, and knowledge helps conquer fear. What steps have you taken to learn enough about your cancer to help alleviate your fears?

I had been battling fear, panic, depression, mood swings, and all the other things that go along with having breast cancer for some women. For a long time I would wake up at about 3:00 A.M. every night. I felt terribly alone, even with my husband lying next to me.

It was at that time that I would have what I refer to as the *big chill*. The fear of a painful death in the not too distant future would overwhelm me. Sometimes I would lie there in the dark and plan my funeral. I would try to think of all the wonderful things that everyone would say about me—how strong I had been . . . what an inspiration I had been . . . how everyone thought I had been very brave, even in the last days . . . and on and on.

When I told my doctor what I was experiencing, he recommended Zoloft. Wow! Now I feel really alive and have hope and a greater feeling of gratitude. I probably should have been on Zoloft years ago. I realize now, after talking with a counselor, that I have been depressed to a greater or lesser degree all my life!

I feel strongly that any woman who is suffering emotionally should not hesitate to tell her doctor and ask for something to help with the fears and anxiety. If Zoloft is not the appropriate medication, something else will work. Because our doctors are frequently focused on the physical aspects of our cancer, we need to be proactive and tell them how we are feeling emotionally and ask for help when we need it.

Les

Do you think you have given your doctor all the information he or she needs to provide you with optimum care, physical and emotional, in treating all aspects of your illness?

I am very thankful to be here to celebrate my fifty-fourth birthday today. Before entering "cancerland," I used to think birthdays were sort of annoying. I mean, who wanted to get older? Right? *Well, I do!*

Now each birthday is a gift for me and for my children. When I was first diagnosed I thought maybe I would not even make it to this birthday. I plan to really celebrate each of my birthdays for a long, long time.

Blair

Do you find you now have a different attitude toward growing older?

I am fortunate. My cancer was diagnosed early and turned out to be very treatable. Even so, it seems to have taken over my life for a while during surgery and recovery, and especially since I am having radiation.

But I was definitely more relaxed after my surgery and when I found out my prognosis. The time between the initial diagnosis and the actual surgery, I think, was the hardest time. Things do get better after you know in more detail what you're dealing with.

A friend who has been through this told me there *will come* a day when I won't worry about breast cancer every day. Right now it's hard not to when I have to run to the hospital for daily radiation treatments. But I have only nine treatments left to go. So there is an end in sight!

Even now, though, the cancer has not completely taken over my life. My life is very full of many wonderful things that have nothing to do with cancer. I have been working full-time as a kindergarten teacher. I planned and carried out a beautiful fiftieth anniversary party for my husband's parents. I got Christmas ready for five boys (three stepsons and two sons). And I have been actively involved in church activities. I have found that many women continue doing all the things they were doing before, in spite of it all. I try to remind myself not to be so busy worrying about dying that I forget to live!

Jan

What has been the worst time for you emotionally in dealing with breast cancer? Do you feel somewhat proud of yourself for making it "through everything"? You should.

I really hate being in chemopause!

I am forty-two and had my periods all during my chemotherapy. Then I started on tamoxifen. Boy!

The hot flashes started immediately. I started sort of studying them. Now I can tell when I'm going to have one because I feel chilly. Then I get really hot, starting in my chest and neck (forget about wearing turtlenecks). Then I get cold again.

It's not so bad. I have not had to ask my doctor for anything to help with the hot flashes. But sometimes I do throw off the covers at night and then, ten minutes later, I'm pulling them all back over me. Oh well!

Leigh

You may have had to make certain adjustments as a result of surgery and/or treatment. Have the adjustments been overwhelming, or have you found them manageable?

I am now facing a bilateral mastectomy/chemo/radiation. I tell myself and I tell others that I want to *live*. If breast cancer is endangering my life, I want the cancer gone; hence, the breasts have to go.

I have said, "My breasts are not vital organs like the heart or lungs." But when they are gone, I know I will definitely mourn my loss. Although they are not large, I have been very happy with them. Now that I am almost fifty-eight years old, they are not as important to me as they once were.

Each situation is unique. This is what I feel comfortable doing. Another woman with what on the surface might appear to be the same diagnosis as mine could make a different decision, and that decision would be right for her. I feel we all need to keep our individual differences in mind when we are talking with each other about diagnosis and treatment.

Do you try to refrain from comparing notes about the specifics of your medical diagnosis and treatment with other breast cancer patients—for your own peace of mind as well as theirs?

I was diagnosed in May and had an MRM. I worried about what my fiancé's reaction would be, but he has been wonderful. I think he is just about the most wonderful man on earth!

He has made the journey much easier. We are planning now to get married in April, a couple of months after I finish chemo. We almost did it before the surgery, but decided to wait until we could enjoy it. It was scary, to say the least, but he held in there for me and I thank God for him every day!

Mary

Who has helped make your journey easier?

When the surgeon told me it was cancer, I turned around to see who she was talking to. There was no one else in the room. "I'm too young to die!" I heard myself say. I had two little ones to take care of: a seven-and-a-half-year-old and an eleven-month-old I was still breast-feeding.

I immediately made provisions for my babies to be taken care of no matter what happens to me. If my husband were to die, their godparents, our best friends, whom the children adore, will take care of them and rear them.

Once I had taken care of these arrangements, I felt a sense of freedom and energy to fight the cancer, with renewed determination to beat it and watch both children graduate from college.

Anita

What have you done for yourself to help ease your mind about the future of the ones you love so that you can work on your own future?

I have a nephew who almost died of leukemia when he was six years old. He and his mother had a daily habit of sitting together in the evening and listing what had been good about the day. As a pastor, I have suggested this as a good first-year practice for newly married couples, but I forgot about it for myself until just now.

Caroline

Try keeping a list of the things you find "good about today."

Hi Newbees,

That's a nickname for you newly diagnosed breast cancer survivors.

I'm involved in active treatment because my breast cancer has metastasized to my lungs, chest, lymph nodes, and some spots in my bones, ribs, etc. The support I receive from my friends is indispensable to me!

The best news is that the new chemo I'm on seems to be working. The last CT scans show a reduction in size of the lesions, nodes, and the mass in the chest! So, in that way, I hope to be an inspiration to all.

I've been around for ten years, and I'm *not* giving up yet! I'll fight as long as I can and do whatever I need to in order to stay around much longer! Hang in there. You can make it, too!

God bless,

Nan

How is your "fighting spirit"?

I have learned a few cosmetic tips that help if you have hair loss. Use eyeliner if you've lost your lashes; eyebrow pencil for brows. Go dark, even if you're blond or *were* blond.

Turbans never worked for me. They made me feel like Norma Desmond on a bad day, and when you don't have any hair under them, they look flat and sort of depressed. At the "Look Good, Feel Better" session I attended, they suggested stuffing turbans with shoulder pads. Falsies for turbans? Could work, although I would worry that the thing could shift under the turban, which could look really weird.

I recommend thrift shops and vintage clothing shops for old hats. Frequently the hats have some structure and style. Some even have a little bit of veil. I wore one, with a wig, to a downtown bar mitzvah. And only a few close friends knew everything on my head was off the rack.

Joyce

Even if you have not lost your hair, you may want to try some new accessories and makeup to give yourself a lift and a fresh and confident feeling about your appearance.

83

My mother was diagnosed four months ago and is undergoing chemotherapy. She lost her hair a couple of months ago and now has a nice wig. Because I live fairly close to her, I have been driving her to her chemo treatments. Sometimes she's a little tense, and I try hard to think of something that will make her laugh.

Last week I took her to her third chemo treatment. It was pouring down rain when we were driving home. We started skidding at one point and we both screamed. We slid off the road and onto the shoulder, almost into a ditch. We were absolutely terrified.

I started checking her to make sure she was okay. Suddenly I yelled, "Mom, you've lost your hair." She looked at me quizzically and said, "I know, dear." I blurted out, "No, I mean your wig is gone." "Oh," she said, "where is it?" We looked everywhere. It was in the back seat.

She quickly slapped it on her head, just as a patrol car pulled up to check on us. We were laughing hysterically. I think the officer thought we were tipsy at three o'clock in the afternoon. We did not try to explain; we just sat there giggling while he radioed for assistance.

Mother and I have been laughing about that afternoon ever since. What a gift of grace humor is during times like these.

Ann

Try to tell a family member or a friend about two things that have made you smile or laugh out loud in the past week.

When I was diagnosed with breast cancer eight years ago, I had a mastectomy and chemotherapy. The treatments went fine, but I was thrown into a depression so deep that I knew I needed help. I was afraid and did not want to go for counseling, but it was the single best thing I have ever done for my mental health.

My counselor showed me that my depression was really a chronic, lifelong illness that had been severely exacerbated by the situation of my having cancer and worrying obsessively. My doctor gave me Prozac, and it helps me tremendously. This past year I was diagnosed with breast cancer for the second time—a new cancer in the other breast. Believe it or not, I am not depressed now.

Having walked in the depression shoes, I understand that one cannot always pull oneself out of it. When you are really depressed, every new blow pulls you down more. True clinical depression is something we usually need help to manage and to move beyond, whether with counseling or medication or both.

Grief is different from depression. It is a very sad but healthy process. Many of us go through a kind of grief process as a part of the breast cancer experience. This is healthy if we can keep moving through the stages and come through to a new understanding and acceptance. But sometimes we get stuck and actually move into depression. There should be no shame in seeking help for this kind of illness any more than in seeking help for cancer. I believe anyone who finds herself barely able or unable to cope should seek help right away.

Mary Lou

Have you ever felt you could no longer cope with everyday life? What did you do to help yourself in response to those feelings?

During my diagnosis and battle with breast cancer, my family has not been very supportive. My mom is losing her six-year battle with cancer. I have three brothers, none of whom came home for Thanksgiving—probably Mom's last. I do feel very alone.

But you can't change how other people treat you, and it is very frustrating to try to get them to change. You have to look for other sources of interaction and support. I may not be able to rely on support from my family, but I do have friends. And I am Christian, and I know Christ is with me always.

Ann

What is your greatest source of comfort and reassurance?

One of my breast cancer friends lost her grandson this year to an accident. When we went to a choral presentation together at Christmastime, she cried all through it. Her tears didn't matter one little bit to me. They gave me a chance to share her grief, hug the daylights out of her, and let her speak about him.

Christmas is a time of joy, but it is also a time to miss those family members who have gone ahead of us. If we are hurting during the holidays, we need to be honest about our feelings and let our friends and family help.

After my mother died, my father gave up holidays for years. It separated him from his children. He is only now beginning to realize that by trying to "spare" everyone (and himself) from the pain of loss at holidays, he merely distanced himself from those who could have shared his sorrow, memories, and hope for the future.

Carol

If you find yourself being sad as the holidays approach, try making everything "new" this year. Rather than using old decorations that are heavy with memories, take a totally new approach.

I have two sons and couldn't bear to think of their future without me. When I found out I had breast cancer, I sat down and wrote letters. I wrote a letter for every event in their life that I felt was important, such as birthdays, graduations, and weddings. It took quite a while, but the sense of accomplishment and relief was incredible.

I gave these letters to my husband to place in a safety-deposit box until the appropriate time. I recommend everyone do this whether or not they have this disease.

You never really know when your time will be up. All you can do is play every hand you are dealt the best you can in this game of life.

Glenda

What provisions do you want to make to be present to those you love, no matter what happens?

I had a lumpectomy in August of 1995, then six months of chemo and eight weeks of radiation. I don't know whether the fear ever goes away. I have talked with women who are twelve to fifteen years post op and still have fears.

But the key is this: Don't let fear rule your life. Let it be there to make you cautious and aware of your body, but don't let it control you. I don't mean to sound like I think I know everything. I'm just saying this to kind of remind myself of the same thing!

Gail

Fear can help us be responsible, but it can also be debilitating. What is your greatest fear, and how do you cope with it?

I am not going to sound like Pollyanna. Cancer is the pits! But breast cancer is one of the few cancers that people actually use the word "cured" about. Although it was the toughest thing I have had to face personally, I have come out stronger, with a new sense of priorities and the knowledge that I am surrounded by love and support—wonderful gifts in the midst of a nightmare.

It is very important to be willing to accept the support and love of others, and to know when it is time to ask for help.

Do you feel "stronger" now than you did before? Do you feel you have matured somewhat emotionally?

The following statement is on a plaque in my radiation oncologist's office. I was going to copy it down. But at my in-laws' fiftieth wedding anniversary, I met a wonderful woman who has been fighting her own battle for years, and she gave it to me on a button.

What cancer *cannot* do . . .

It cannot cripple love, shatter hope, corrode faith, destroy peace, kill friendship, suppress memories, silence courage, invade the soul, steal eternal life, or conquer the spirit.

Jan

Do you sometimes feel your disease has ruined everything important to you? Try to make a list of all the intangible and wonderful things in your life that cancer cannot touch.

I have found that I have to be very assertive and often blunt with my friends. I have one friend who was determined to see only the worst scenarios and smother me with caring. While I know she wanted only the best, it drove me crazy!

I finally told her what I needed and how I was choosing to deal with this whole thing. I carried it one step further and told her that if she could not help me in these areas, then I needed not to visit with her. Telling her this was difficult, and she continued doing some of the same things, but at a much reduced level that we both could handle.

I have found people have a hard time dealing with cancer in general, and especially breast cancer. Sometimes they say the strangest things, things that really hurt. Then I find myself dwelling on what they have said that upset me.

To help me get past some of that, I think about our conversation and usually realize the person didn't say it intentionally. It was their way of trying to help, even if they missed the mark. The other side is they are describing what they think might help them, but that doesn't necessarily help me. It is done with the right intention, but the execution is faulty. That enables me to "forgive" and move on.

I also found that my friends and family respond in very different ways. Some are better support for some parts of the journey than others are.

Marcia

Can you determine who among your friends and family are good at a specific kind of support? How is your mother, father, or sibling different from your best friend or lover in such situations?

I was diagnosed with breast cancer on July 9 this year. They did a needle biopsy and lumpectomy on August 1. On August 9, I had a partial mastectomy done, and twelve lymph nodes were removed. Two out of the twelve nodes were cancerous. It was determined that I had stage II breast cancer.

I started intense chemotherapy September 7, on my thirty-seventh wedding anniversary. I was scheduled for four treatments, twenty-one days apart. I finished my treatments on November 8 without too much trouble.

On November 26, I found another lump on the same breast. I had three doctors look at it, and they all agreed that it was nothing to worry about. I will take their word for it, not just because they are the specialists, but because I trust and respect them. I will be starting my radiation treatments tomorrow. I should finish them January 20, six days before my fifty-seventh birthday. Then I will be on tamoxifen for five years.

I have had the best support from my very wonderful husband. My sons and daughters-in-law have been great, and the rest of my family and friends have been there for me—even friends I didn't know I had. I think now that this illness has been a blessing for me in that I appreciate my family and friends more now than ever, and I am trying to make sure to live each day to the fullest.

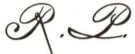

You probably respect your doctors, but do you ever have difficulty relaxing and trusting them because of your own doubts and fears? How do you distinguish when it is appropriate to question and when you need to let go of trying to "second guess"? Do you find second opinions helpful?

I had an MRM and tram flap last month. Although I've had some bad moments (especially the first couple of days after surgery), on the whole I've really felt pretty upbeat. All the news I've had—except, of course, for the fact that I've got breast cancer—has been good. I'm recovering from surgery much better than I had anticipated, and my friends have been incredible.

Then yesterday I go to my plastic surgeon. Fortunately he takes out my last drains, takes off the huge bandages around my new appendage, and tells me I can shower, which I've been dreaming about.

So everything's going just great, and I'm just sailing along. I go into the bathroom and take off my bandages for my shower. Then I look at myself in the mirror and just lose it. I bawl and bawl. I just can't stop crying. My poor husband, Len, opens the door and asks what's wrong, and all I can say is that I have just looked at myself for the first time.

I guess he decides he should leave and get the kids ready for school and keep them away from me, which is probably a good idea, but that is not necessarily what I need. I feel like I've got the creature that ate Milwaukee on my chest. I know it will get better, but I cannot be comforted by that thought.

I guess maybe this is the first time I've really started to deal with what has happened to me. Now I am starting to go through some of the grieving process. Anyway, I know it will be better tomorrow. And I do have this new streamlined tummy.

Jan

Sometimes it is hard to see a good tomorrow in the fears and disappointments of today. In what areas of your life are you having to "be on hold" and try to convince yourself that the future joys will make today's pain worthwhile?

Right before Christmas in 1996, after I had my mastectomy and before I began the chemotherapy, a friend gave me a very large, heavy gift bag—the type with a rope handle and a pretty, glossy Christmas picture on both sides. She said it was filled with all kinds of little gifts that were individually wrapped. I was instructed to dip into it whenever I felt particularly depressed or blue.

I have opened many of the gifts and there seems to be no end to the gifts in the bag. Some of the gifts have been hand lotion, Christmas ornaments, a small box of graham crackers, a Barbie coloring book with crayons, a Christmas hand towel, and a paperback book on Barbra Streisand (my friend knows I like her singing). I have opened many more, but I can't think what they all are right now.

This was a very thoughtful gift. My friend has had a lot of physical and emotional problems, and she knows what it is like to cope with feeling down. It is so nice when I dip into the bag and realize I deserve a little reward and pick-me-up. It also calls to mind how thoughtful and caring my friend is.

Carol

Do you know someone who needs a bag of thoughtful surprises?

The fear of breast cancer can take over your life if you let it! The period of time between diagnosis and knowing what lies ahead in terms of prognosis and treatment may seem to be a black hole—a time when you have only fear and no real answers. I've been on this roller coaster for ten years, and most of those ten years have been wonderful! I did all the things I wanted to do when we lived in Hawaii—camping, swimming, bowling in tournaments, golfing, learning to enjoy my husband and my family a whole lot more!

When we moved here to Virginia, right after my husband retired from the military, we had no idea what he would do as a civilian. That was really scary—no home, no jobs, a thirteen-year-old and an unmarried eighteen-year-old daughter with a two-month-old son! As usual, God took care of us. The jobs materialized, as well as the homes to rent and eventually buy.

My breast cancer first recurred at the five-year mark and then again at the ten-year mark (mets to lungs, lymph nodes, and bones). But in the last few years, I've really gotten to know and learned to love my four grandchildren, my wonderful daughter-in-law, and my own kids as they've grown up to be wonderful adults. And I have learned to love and better appreciate this wonderful man I married who has stuck by me for thirty-one years and who has put up with so much from me!

Right now breast cancer has again taken over my life, even more so than ever before because it is more serious this time. If I can get beyond the active treatments into a treatment-free time, I hope to have the strength and energy to *do something* with the rest of my life—something to make a difference in this world! If I *can't* ever get beyond monthly chemo and tests, etc., then I hope and pray God will help me to live out these next years more gracefully than I feel I do right now. I do put my trust and faith in God to help guide others and me along the way!

All things considered, breast cancer is one of the easier diseases to treat, and surprisingly, it can bring many blessings!

Nan

What are the two main things you want to do with the rest of your life?

I'm a survivor of more than a decade. Rather than have the second breast removed, I had reconstruction. The plastic surgeon recommended also putting a silicone implant in the second breast because he could better match the two sides.

I happened to be one of those few people who had lots of problems with implants. Now I wish someone had just advised me to have surgery on both sides and that I had forgone the implants. But hindsight is 20/20, and if I had had a bilateral I might always feel I had cheated myself.

Bets

How do you feel personally when you consider that we must simply make the best decisions we can with the information available to us at the time?

I read somewhere that the very act of smiling, even when you are alone, will release endorphins and make the moment more enjoyable. Don't just smile with your mouth when you try this, also use your eyes. Make it an "authentic" smile.

When you're not sure whether your smile is authentic, look in the mirror and check yourself and your smile. It sounds simple, but it works.

Begin with the smiling facial expression, and the happy emotion will follow. I have tried it and confidently recommend it as a mood brightener.

Lee

When you are feeling low, how do you help yourself feel more cheerful?

There are some days I need sugarcoated messages. I was diagnosed with breast cancer in April 1995 and am now watching a forty-two-year-old cousin fight stage IV breast cancer.

I feel I am an intelligent woman, and I know a lot about my disease. I know a lot about treatments, and I have wonderful doctors. But there are times when I just need sugarcoated messages, times when I don't want to deal with all the implications of my disease and possibilities for the future.

It's like those days when things are going crazy at work and I wish I could be home and get a hug from my hubby. It might not change things, but it sure helps. So do smiles and laughter. I certainly enjoy my friends, some of whom are survivors. We get together and laugh and have a great time. Sometimes we do talk about health issues, but sometimes we just play. I can see their smiles and hear their laughter always with me. I am so glad I have them.

Nancy

Try to "cut yourself some slack." Do you give yourself permission to be comforted by "sugarcoated" messages and platitudes?

In May I had an MRM and I am still on chemo. In October, with the help of people at work, I presented four half-hour sessions on the signs and symptoms of breast cancer.

I found it to be very helpful for me and my recovery. I know several women who decided to get checkups and mammograms. Some of the men in my office passed the information on to their wives. If I helped others to avoid some the challenges I have had to face, then the talks were a success.

Mary

Are there ways you can help yourself by helping others?

Keeping a journal can be very helpful in the present and later when you want to look back and see how far you've come. With the right speaker, this can be a great support group topic.

Two years ago our group invited an English instructor to speak on journaling. It drew so much interest that she held a couple of workshops, and a lot of women in our group started keeping a journal. A few of us have been keeping journals for the entire two years.

Occasionally when we share entries, we can see tremendous progress and a shift in priorities to what is really important in our lives. This in itself has given a real boost to lots of our recently diagnosed women. They can see that others had similar feelings at diagnosis, and then they can see that those women have not only survived but have found that there *is* good life after breast cancer.

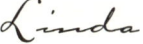

If you don't already keep a journal, try keeping one for the next six weeks. At the end of that time, look back at your first few entries. You will probably find them interesting and will begin to appreciate the value of recording your thoughts and feelings on a regular basis.

I have stage IV breast cancer with mets to the bone. My oncologist recommended HDC/SCR (high-dose chemotherapy/stem cell recovery). At first I was afraid to do it. It is a relatively new procedure and is frequently effective at putting stage IV patients who qualify for the procedure into remission.

It usually requires hospitalization until your blood counts are high enough to avoid the risk of infection, about three to six weeks; however, some hospitals are starting to experiment with doing it on an outpatient basis. They determine whether you are eligible based on whether you are sufficiently responsive to chemo and whether your "tumor" load is low enough that they think they can "get it all" with the high-dose chemo.

For the past year I've been trying to get my tumor load low enough to go ahead. Finally I am there, and I have just completed my second day of pheresis to harvest my stem cells. Everything went really well. Now I get to lie low for two weeks prior to the HDC and reinfusion of the stem cells.

This technology is really wonderful. I must admit that I'm not on top of the world, but it really hasn't been that bad for me. I was encouraged when a friend of mine made the following suggestions for my hospital stay: Take lots of stuff to do in the hospital, like books, magazines, Walkman, music tapes, inspirational tapes, writing paper, address book, and phone book. At times you may not feel like doing much of this, but if you are feeling pretty good, you'll be glad you brought things to keep you busy. Also take your diary/journal. I look back at mine sometimes for a lot of different reasons.

Actually, I'm grateful to have the opportunity to have this treatment, and I am looking forward to a *long* remission.

Adrienne

When you start thinking about "the worst that could happen," try to consider the strides that are being made today in the treatment of breast cancer.

Fortunately, I have been able to come through my own battle with this disease. My mother died of breast cancer and I miss her terribly, but there is no one to blame for her death—not her, not me, not God. The same principle applies to my trying to sort out why I got breast cancer. I know I cannot and should not blame her death or myself or my attitude or God for my breast cancer.

After struggling to sort all this out, I now understand that these things just happen to us as a part of life. Fortunately God is with us as we go through our daily struggles. And God is always with each of us, even in death.

Death for my mother came much too early (she was only fifty-two), but death is a part of life. I teach school, and the following is an excerpt from *The Velveteen Rabbit* that I recently read to the students in my class:

"What is REAL?" asked the Rabbit one day, when he and the Skin Horse were lying side by side near the nursery fender, before Nana came to tidy the room. "Does it mean having things that buzz inside you and a stick-out handle?"

"Real isn't how you are made," said the Skin Horse. "It's a thing that happens to you. When a child loves you for a long, long time, not just to play with, but REALLY loves you, then you become Real."

"Does it hurt?" asked the Rabbit.

"Sometimes," said the Skin Horse, for he was always truthful. "When you are Real you don't mind being hurt."

"Does it happen all at once, like being wound up," he asked, "or bit by bit?"

"It doesn't happen all at once," said the Skin Horse. "You become. It takes a long time. That's why it doesn't often happen to people who break easily, or have sharp edges, or who have to be carefully kept. Generally, by the time you are Real, most of your hair has been loved off, and your eyes drop out and you get loose in the joints and very shabby. But these things don't matter at all, because once you are Real, you can't be ugly, except to people who don't understand."

For me *The Velveteen Rabbit* is also a resurrection story. I am reassured that God is with all of us, that God does everything possible for us. No matter what happens, we will all "become real" someday.

Jan

What does becoming real mean to you?

Choices are just that—choices.
Each one is very personal. Each choice you make comes out of your individual past and present—who you are, where you've come from, where you are in your life right now.

My breast surgeon didn't think the mastectomy was necessary, but the radiation oncologist agreed with me that I should have one. Having lost a twelve-year-old to leukemia thirteen years ago, I wanted to give my surviving eighteen-year-old daughter the best chance possible of having her mom with her.

I hope I made the "right choice" (if there is such a thing), but I've never regretted the decision I made. I fervently hope that *all* of us who are survivors can have peace of mind and heart—and longevity, too.

Lenore

How do you feel about the decisions regarding your course of treatment? Is there anything you would like to discuss further with your doctor(s)?

My original diagnosis of breast cancer was when I was twenty-four, with a recurrence and metastasis to both lungs at twenty-six. I remember looking at my chest X-ray and seeing all the tumors the radiologist had marked and thinking, "Those can't possibly be my lungs."

I then had a year of chemo. Since then I have enjoyed a twelve-year remission! All of us who are survivors need to pray for ourselves and for each other. We need to trust in God and spit in cancer's eye (figure of speech).

Janice

How do you think your attitude and your spiritual life affect your illness and your whole self?

A friend of mine went for a biopsy the other day and called me to talk about how scared she was, since she knows I have already been down the breast cancer road. I told her women don't die from cancer of the breast; they die from cancer that has spread from their breast to other parts of their body, and this takes time. If there is a malignancy, finding and treating it early is the key to a long and happy life.

I reminded her not to panic but to stay cool and to stay informed, and not to try to anticipate what's coming—just take it one step at a time.

These same principles apply to those of us "on the other side of the experience," especially when something new or different crops up. We have to relearn and sometimes relive how to deal with those first moments of uncertainty, but for me that has never been as bad as the first time around.

Catherine

Do you have your own list of things to quiet you when you do become anxious? What kinds of things are helpful to you?

My mom died a few years after my initial diagnosis and treatment. I was the one who had to empty my mom's house and put it up for sale. I also arranged yard sales to dispose of what we three kids didn't want. Actually, although it was work, and although I cried a lot, it was very good for me in helping me resolve a few remaining issues in our relationship.

Daily I talked to her, scolding her for not letting me use certain fabrics thirty years ago, because I was finding them still packed away unused and rotten! I got to yell at her, sleep in her bed at night, and feel comforted. I got to box up her jams and jellies for our families to enjoy. And I was able just to grieve for her in a very healing way.

Here it is eight years later, and there are times when I just yearn to talk to her. We were pretty good friends, and I am amazed she is gone. But I've gotten beyond the heartbreak into the fond memories.

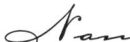

Have you ever found that "good grieving" helps you move to a new place in your relationship with a loved one who has died?

I have found the following helpful in my adult life but especially during my experience with breast cancer. Someone gave me this list and I refer to it often:

- ❖ Do you ever find yourself putting yourself down either aloud or in your thoughts? When you catch yourself, try to stop the negative thought and reword it as a positive thought.

- ❖ Are you more critical of yourself than you are of others? If so, why? Try to reframe your thoughts in such a way that you will be able to view yourself in a more positive and forgiving light.

- ❖ When someone praises you or shows you gratitude, can you say thank you? Try to allow yourself to feel the other person's appreciation.

- ❖ Most important, give yourself credit for the nice things you do or have done for others.

These exercises have helped me understand that to a certain extent I can have some control over how I feel about myself *and* that I should not shortchange myself.

Jennifer

How you feel about yourself can affect every aspect of your mental and physical well-being. What measures are you taking to be realistic and supportive of your image of yourself?

At the end of chemo and/or radiation treatments, we frequently enter a period of reflection.

Some of my well-meaning friends said things like, "Well, aren't you glad it's all over now and you can get on with your life as usual?" Well, for me it was not as easy as that. I was tired for a period of time after radiation and chemo, and I found I needed a while to reflect on what had occurred in my life.

I concentrated very hard on returning to "normal," but it was hard to put it all behind me. I had my last treatment eighteen months ago, but I still worry, even now. I don't dwell on it, but I try to be realistic and honest with myself. I've decided that nothing we feel is wrong or weird. We have all been there and are still going through it, each with her own unique reactions.

E. R.

What feelings are you acutely aware of at this time?

Knowledge is power and igno-rance *is not* bliss! *Not knowing* is *always* worse than knowing, don't you think? Once you *know* your enemy or your disease, you can deal with it. You may not be able to change it, but a lot of the weight of the fear is gone!

I have mets to the lung and bone. I keep copies of *all* my labs, tests, scans, etc. I carry them with me from doctor to doctor, so each doctor can check back and get anything he or she needs *and* so that I'm not a "nervous Nellie," sitting there quaking in my boots! I've learned a *lot* during the past ten years on this breast cancer road.

Each of us needs to do whatever is best for her. Not everyone can or wants to handle this kind of knowledge. For me, it is the only way I feel I have a semblance of control—even though I know I don't ultimately have any control over my situation. At least I can talk and listen intelligently when I'm around the doctors and nurses.

Because I know God has absolute control over my life and my death, I guess when all is said and done, I must accept whatever comes along. But by keeping myself knowledgeable about num-bers or symptoms, I have been able to actively participate with my doctors in my treatments. I feel this is one way I can keep up *my* part of this partnership!

Nan

In what ways do you actively participate with your doctors in your care?

To my friends on the breast cancer message board:

Hi there. I'm still down, but not yet out, as you can tell!

It's a blessing that I can wake up every day and see the sun come up and go down again. It's amazing how I'm noticing more of what is around me now that I have the time to "stop and smell the roses."

One Christmas wish I have is to see snow. Not very likely in Portland, Oregon, but I can always dream! My other wish is for all of you that have been in contact with me through this message board: May your lives be filled with happiness and may you enjoy each day. You have all blessed my life, and I feel very lucky to have spent time on this board and to have listened to you all.

Thank you for your prayers and love. You are all in my thoughts this holiday season. By the way, for those of you who know me, the doctors are still wrong—I'm still here!

Talk to you all soon! Let me know if you are going to have any online chats in the next few days. I would love to try to join in!

What do you think is the relationship between serenity and courage? Whom do you know who is especially courageous and/or serene?

My mother died of breast cancer that had metastasized to the bone. It was a very tough time for me because my first marriage was falling apart as well. Even though it was normal to grieve the way I did, I found counseling to be very helpful. Grief work takes an incredibly long time. The first year is especially hard during the holidays. My mother died twelve years ago, but there are still times I miss her terribly.

I have to say that one positive thing that has happened to me in the midst of grief and my breast cancer is that I have developed some valuable personal resources that have helped me deal with the cancer. I know I have grown a lot since my mother died. If I hadn't I wouldn't be able to cope now.

Counseling is not the answer for everyone, but we all need someone at times, and often the people closest to us cannot be that someone because they are going through their own "stuff." When you go to a counselor, you have a safe place to dump all the emotions you are dealing with, and it can lead to tremendous personal growth.

Jan

Do you sometimes feel the need to vent, complain, or just talk about your situation with *someone else*—someone other than your closest family and friends?

I am a single mom and had my MRM at Christmastime last year. A friend of mine took her kids and mine to see Santa. She told me my two girls (ages five and seven) climbed onto Santa's lap, and in their small voices she heard them say, "Our mommy has cancer. Will you make her well?"

My friend said she nearly burst into tears. Santa offered to pray for me and looked at her with tears in his eyes. Then he said a prayer right then and there!

Gail

In what kinds of unexpected ways have you found support and comfort?

Six years ago when I was first diagnosed and had a mastectomy and chemo, I attended a small support group for breast cancer patients. Many of the women were there to discuss reconstructive surgery, but some of us talked about our worst fears and what it was like to be on chemotherapy.

I particularly remember one young woman named Ginger. She had just had surgery and was starting her chemotherapy. Her oncologist had advised her to purchase a wig because with the chemo she was receiving, she would almost certainly lose all her hair.

She had beautiful red hair, and she showed us her new wig. She vowed that once she lost her hair she would wear her wig all the time, day and night. She said she never wanted anyone to see her without her "hair." She didn't even want to see herself in the mirror without hair.

A couple of months later she came to the meeting with a hat on and no wig underneath. No one commented on it, but when it came her time to share she said, "I lost my hair last month." We nodded. "You know how I said I would always wear my wig." We nodded. "Well, it's August, and yesterday I was about to burn up. My wig was really uncomfortable, and I decided that with all I've been through and am now going through I wanted to be comfortable, not miserable with artificial hair. Anyway, it will grow back eventually."

We all need ways to cope with each new challenge, large or small. Sometimes we will make promises to ourselves based on our current pressing needs. These temporary coping mechanisms serve us well while we need them. Later, however, when we have a new perspective, we are frequently able to abandon these ways of coping.

Lee

Have you made any declarations to help you get through a rough spot that you later were able to give up? How did they help you?

I was nicely wigged and dressed to a T. I had tried to glue on false eyelashes, but gave up when I realized I looked like Tammy Faye. My husband and I were entertaining good friends, and it was the first time I had tried to cook a large meal with my wig on.

I worked hard over the oven, and I presented a tasty meal that everyone enjoyed. Our friends were happy, and we all had a great time. Just before dessert, I stepped into the bathroom and looked in the mirror. I gasped. The entire front of my wig was a solid melted glob. Obviously I had gotten a bit too close when checking the roast. I couldn't believe no one had said a word! They were trying to spare *me* the embarrassment.

I walked back into the dining room laughing so hard I could hardly stand up. The laughter was contagious, and before long everyone was in stitches. This laughter led us all into the first heart-to-heart conversation we had had since my diagnosis. The tears, shed in humor, opened the doors to sharing the pain. The shields went down and hearts connected. Thank God for giving us the gift of humor!

Tracy

Has humor broken down any barriers for you?

This morning I drove my thirteen-year-old daughter to school. I have been housebound since August (with the exception of going to radiation treatments and doctors' appointments) because of bone mets to the spine and neck.

I am finally better, and now I can drive. My daughter's ride couldn't take her this morning. Just being able to get into the car and go out on a crisp, sunny morning was a pleasure. It is indeed a beautiful day.

Joyce

What victories large or small have you experienced during your diagnosis and treatment?

I was diagnosed and had surgery in March of 1993. I can remember thinking, *I hope I can make it to next Christmas.*

I mentioned this to a friend one day, and she retorted, "Not only will you make it to Christmas, but there's your February birthday, and Easter after that. And don't forget Memorial Day, Fourth of July, Halloween, Thanksgiving, and the next Christmas."

There are no constraints on any of us. God watches over us and blesses us each day.

Mary Margaret

How do you go about making holidays special for you personally and for your family and friends?

I received my diagnosis in August of 1995, had a lumpectomy, chemo, and radiation, and now I am doing *great*! There a few hints I found very useful in dealing with my doctors when I was first diagnosed. Dr. Susan Love's *Breast Book* helped me know what questions to ask my surgeon. I also found it helpful to write all my questions down, right when I was thinking of them.

Sometimes on my doctor visits I would be nervous and couldn't keep everything the doctor said all straight. I tried to take someone with me when I went to the doctor to be my extra ears and eyes and help me interpret later exactly what the doctor had said. But I also wanted someone there to lend moral support. Sometimes I took a tape recorder to my doctor visits. Also, I think it is always a good idea to ask for a second opinion. Most insurance companies cover it.

Gail

Do you have any learnings or suggestions you would like to pass on to other women that would help them during their treatment?

I am an only child, and I didn't want my mother to be with me during my surgery and treatment. In fact, I realized I needed *not* to tell her, because this was a time when she should not be allowed to come in and "take over" as she has done all my life.

If I had interacted with her during my treatment, everything would have been all about her, centered around her needs and fears. Anything that happens to me immediately becomes her problem, and she tries to become the center of everyone's attention. Usually I just go along with her behavior and wait for her to "get over it."

But this was a time when I knew I had to focus on taking care of myself. I didn't need to start having to take care of my mother and dealing with how bad she felt. My mother means well, but she was raised to be self-centered and it worked!

When I had finished my chemo, I called her and gently told her what was going on—that I am fine and that I love her and didn't want to cause her unnecessary worry. She was upset, but she got calmed down in about a week, and I am planning to fly out to see her next month. I know now that this was the best way to handle the situation. I am glad I finally had the courage to consider my own needs first when it was appropriate to do so.

Holly

Sometimes a crisis of illness exacerbates family conflict. If you have experienced this, how have you handled the situation?

When I was first diagnosed, many people I knew came up with the old cliché "Well, any one of us could step in front of a truck tomorrow." I feel my particular prognosis is not wonderful. I finally had to walk away from one longtime friend who kept insisting that a positive attitude would save my life. She just didn't get the negative implication of that stupid statement.

To say something like this can really put a woman with breast cancer on an unnecessary and unfair guilt trip. "What did I do wrong that made me get breast cancer? Why can't I be cured? Is it lack of faith, the wrong outlook, a sometimes less than positive attitude, something I did when I was young—or something I didn't do?"

Some people don't realize how outrageous it is to blame the patient for getting breast cancer in the first place and then telling her it is somehow her fault if she fails to get well. I think that because some people have not yet come to terms with their own mortality, they feel they must have a reason that things like breast cancer can happen to someone close to them.

Such people feel vulnerable and cast about looking for something or someone to blame in order to keep their own fears at bay. Then they can pretend nothing like this will ever happen to them. With all the literature out today on the relationship between emotions and disease, these folk can take a rather superficial view and blame the easiest target—the breast cancer patient herself. I have to say "No thanks!" to this interpretation of my situation.

Eve

Have you ever felt it might somehow be your fault you have breast cancer? If so, how have you dealt with these feelings? Sometimes it helps to talk them through with your doctor or a caring loved one.

I turned the big "5-0" last month and threw a huge party to celebrate. I invited all my friends and family, and they filled the room with lots of love.

You know, I don't think I would ever have thrown a party for myself before my diagnosis of breast cancer. I would have been reluctant to draw attention to myself.

I now take to heart all those platitudes about life that I once thought were so corny: "Life's too short," "All you need is love," "Live life to the fullest."

Margaret

How have you reached out in joy to those who mean the most to you?

Statistics can be scary, especially if you don't know how what you are looking at or hearing applies to your own situation. I find I can handle only some of them.

This is one of the areas where I no longer seek out information, because it can be so frightening. Also, I figure not having that information will not cause me a problem. For me, it is one less problem to deal with.

Mary

Have you been able to give yourself permission not to listen to people or media presentations that have the potential to cause you anxiety?

I am a breast cancer survivor. I had a lumpectomy in July of 1995 and then radiation. Somehow we do manage to get through this ordeal even though we may think at first it will be impossible.

I got through it because I felt I had to be strong for my ten-year-old daughter. If I let her see me fall apart when something like this happens, how will she be able to handle a problem that comes up in her life someday? I knew I had to be strong for her.

I suppose I have matured somewhat during this experience. I realized for the first time the other day that the word *cancer* doesn't scare me the way it used to, and it doesn't scare my daughter anymore either.

Millie

What elements of your life are so important to you that they lead you to be braver than you think you might otherwise be?

I didn't have reconstruction for a couple of reasons. I had already had a tummy tuck thirteen years ago to repair the damage of thirteen-pound twins, so I didn't have any tummy to borrow from. Also, my natural breasts were so perky and pretty I knew surgery couldn't replace them in my mind. In fact, they were perky because of dense fibrous tissue that masked my tumor so that it didn't show up on the mammogram!

With my sense of humor, I thought I might just have tattoos instead of breasts. Maybe headlights or owls. Then I could show people my hooters!

I applaud every woman who has had to go through this ordeal. If you want breasts, great! If it doesn't matter to you, fine! To each her own decision.

J.F.

How would you characterize your feelings about your natural breasts?

I was diagnosed seven years ago and had an MRM and chemo. I tried to be very careful about checking for recurrence, but in reality I was consumed with fear of recurrence.

About two years after my diagnosis, I had a strange but funny experience. I was showering one morning and discovered a small, hard knot under my left arm, the side of my surgery. Well, I panicked.

I called immediately for an appointment with my oncologist, which is, of course, what I should have done. I set up an appointment for the next day.

My doctor examined the "lump." Then I saw a little smile on her face. When I asked her what she thought, she said, "We don't see this very often, but when we do we always know exactly what it is." She continued, "You're fine. You have an irritated hair follicle, probably as a result of putting on your deodorant right after showering."

I nearly fell over. I laugh about that now every time I think about it.

Kirsten

What new and amusing bits of trivia have you learned in the process of dealing with breast cancer?

I try to enjoy something new each day. We moved into our first "permanent" home this past spring. Until then, it was a new home every two years (except for four years in Japan), compliments of the military. We found a home in north Virginia, on six acres, with a small pond outside our bedroom and living room.

I miss having close neighbors and borrowing a cup of sugar, but my husband loves having the land around us. Just when I start to wonder why the "neighbors" haven't come by with a welcoming casserole, geese will land on the pond, honking and causing our dogs to stand at attention. Mallards and wood ducks also paddle around and search for the corn I throw out. Herons and the smaller cranes land first thing in the morning and are gone by the time the pushy geese arrive.

The many deer (including twins born in my newly established rose bushes) retreat to the woods for the day, only to return around five o'clock to nibble on what is left of my garden. Squirrels knock on our back door for peanuts, and many kinds of birds fill the feeders.

I think my husband had an ulterior motive for wanting this house . . . a place for us to forget about stress. It's hard to believe that ten minutes away is the rest of the world—his work and my doctors. This has to be one of our real blessings.

Millie

In what ways have you actively sought to relieve stress in your life?

I brought home a statuette called a *Daruma* from Japan when we moved back to the States. We had lived in Japan for four years. This *Daruma* is round like a ball and painted the traditional red for New Year's with two big white spots for eyes.

What you do with a *Daruma* is paint a black dot in one of the white spots, thereby giving it one "eye." Then you promise that if the *Daruma* grants your wish, you will paint in its other eye. That was in 1982, also the year of my diagnosis and treatment, and that little sucker still has only one eye!

I can't tell you the wish, but it has something to do with a girlish figure again. The *Daruma* sits in our den, watching the entire family "world" go by. And it still gives me pleasure, because I'm still here and plan to be for a long time.

Millie

Try selecting a tangible object that has some meaning for you in terms of your being a survivor. Place it where it can serve as a constant reminder of how far you've come.

I was almost forty years old when I was diagnosed. I was working out of town on a consultation. I recall going to the public restroom at the hotel. Later in the day I noticed the center stone was missing from a ring my mother had given me. I panicked. This was four hours later. I rushed to the restroom and found the stone against the wall under the towel cabinet. What a relief!

That started my evening. My friend and I went to dinner, then she came to my room to stitch. It had been a long day but a good one; however, my real journey was about to begin.

As I prepared for bed my right hand brushed the upper inside part of my left breast. There was something there about the size of a large egg. What could it be? I checked last month and there was no such thing there! *Cancer can't blow up like this,* I thought to myself.

When I returned to Dallas, my gynecologist referred me to a surgeon, who did a needle biopsy in her office. I was at work when she called to tell me the results were positive. I called my fiancé to tell him and to let him know I wanted him to go with me to my doctor's appointment on Monday.

That weekend was the hardest two days of my life. After I saw the doctor on Monday and she outlined my options for treatment, I began to feel better immediately.

The treatment and recovery were not nearly as bad as I antici-pated, and now, three years later, I feel confident and at peace.

Evelyn

What events do you recall surrounding your diagnosis? In what ways do you feel different now from the way you felt initially?

Friday, March 3, 1995, 2:00 p.m.

Alice and I go into the doctor's office. I have my questions on paper along with fears in my heart and soul. The doctor asks about my questions, but I ask her to tell me what she thinks first. She tells me this is an aggressive tumor and too large for a lumpectomy.

Alice and I want to discuss the course of surgery and treatment. Alice is firm in encouraging the MRM. Then we call the surgeon back with our decision and schedule the surgery for a week from today.

We decide we will live our lives as planned until the surgery next week. We will go to the coast and we will enjoy this final week of my whole physical self. And we decide we will go ahead and buy the house we love so much.

Alice is kind and strong, and I know she will not let me sink into pity and depression. This will be a tough road, and I will need lots of support for a while. I will tell all my friends. Some of the people I work with will get the specifics, some will just know it is a medical emergency.

I now have a deep and nurturing sense that one way or another everything will be okay. I will not lose Alice and I probably won't lose my life. And now to sleep.

Mary Ann

Who was your greatest support during your decision-making process?
How have you expressed your gratitude?

I had an MRM in July of 1996. I began chemotherapy on August 7 and completed chemo in March of 1997.

What I remember most is the unexpected: I lost my nose hairs, and that complicated my allergies. I had to carry a tissue with me at all times.

I remember that the drainage tubes came out in one big pull from the doctor. He warned me of a hollow feeling. He was right. It did feel weird and hollow for a short time. The tubes were the hardest part of the surgical recovery for me. I am sure the fact that I dropped one after my first shower contributed to my uneasiness about them.

During the hardest part of my recovery, adriamycin chemotherapy, I regularly wrote in my journal. This journal has been preserving and soul-saving for me. I always try to note at least five things I am grateful for each day. Some days it is hard, but it does get easier with time.

The best part of it all was that I began looking at things from a very different perspective. I realized that even with the recent turn of events there was a lot to be grateful for. There always had been, but I had been failing to notice.

Marie

Many survivors find their perspective changes during diagnosis and treatment. In what new ways do you look at life now?